My Dyslexic Journey

Sarah Todd

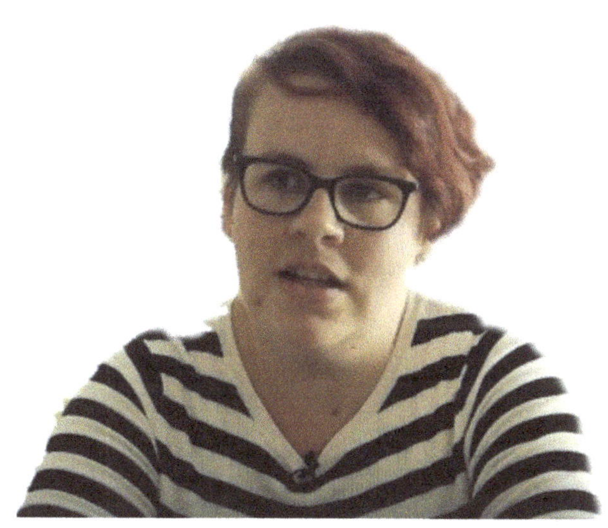

First published in the United Kingdom in 2019
by the Cloister House Press

ISBN 978-1-909465-99-2

Introduction

Today I am sitting in the library reading a fantastic book called "The Other Side of You". I was given this book and three others as a gift, well, reward, for all my hard work and achievement.

In the last three years the other side of **Me** has finally blossomed. I have learnt to read and understand letters and emails. I struggle sometimes but I have the confidence to ask for help and I enjoy reading stories to my twins. It is the best feeling as a parent to be able to sit and read to your children.

Before if you had asked me to read a menu or go to the library I would have given you attitude or changed the subject very quickly. The thought of telling someone I couldn't read because I had dyslexia – yes, the word that explained so much – or admitting I had a problem, was a massive issue for me. I'd rather sit in silence than admit I needed help.

There was a time I would panic or change the subject when it came to reading to my twins. The words, "Mummy, can we have a story?" or "Mummy, what does this say?" would make me sweat and feel sick. I have always struggled but to deny your own children a chance to hear you read to them or teach them something new was heart wrenching. I always felt so annoyed and frustrated - why couldn't I just get the words out and stop panicking?

Today I love being able to offer to read something out loud. I'll read a menu and a paper and instructions or learn something new through words in a book or online.

My twins are doing really well with their reading too which makes me so proud. I enjoy listening as well as reading to them and I know they don't judge me, they just love me.

So how did I get from there to here?

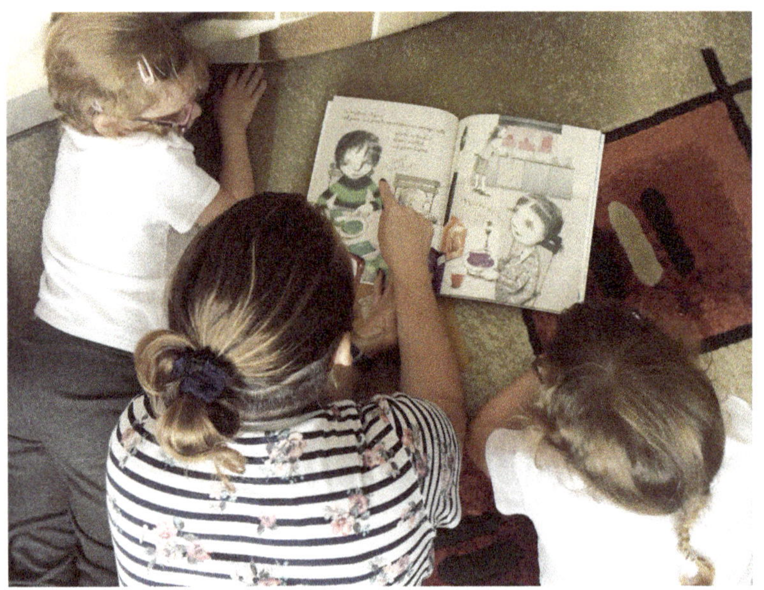

Chapter 1

To base camp and beyond

Reading and writing is supposed to just happen in primary school, isn't it? Well, it didn't quite work that way for me.

The problems started in the first year when I was often sick and off school. This was just as I should have been getting the basics of phonics and word recognition. When I was offered Biff and Chip books on my return I tried reading them but I really couldn't get my head around the words. Instead I would make them up as I went along. I felt very confused. Why didn't the teacher say something or try to encourage me? Why didn't she suggest I started from the beginning with My First Words books or bring to the school's attention that I was in serious need of help?

I was put in a massive classroom filled with dust particles and climbing equipment to avoid being distracted. I still found myself day dreaming instead of concentrating but it was easier because I didn't feel so sad that I couldn't read the words on the page.

During lessons there would be the children who would sit and doodle, the children who would be at the teacher's side and the children who would be reading. I was desperate to be one of the readers and know what the other children were talking about. I wished that somehow one morning I would wake up and be able to read like the others, understand what the teacher was talking about and even read out loud in front of other pupils.

When I was at home I would sit on my bed determined to

read the words on the pages of books I owned. I didn't have many. I would try desperately not to let my mind wander off and make my own stories up. I'd say "Come on, Sarah, just read the words, they are there in front of you. Just read them!" I would get so angry I'd cry and give up.

Chapter 2

Setting out

As I started middle school I was terrified for so many reasons: new teachers, new routines, new kids, even new smells. I struggled to fit in. I was the odd kid who only just knew how to spell her name, couldn't tell the time and couldn't read. School was rubbish and that was the start of my anxiety and depression.

The kids were brutal. "She can't read, she must be stupid." "Look, there goes the spastic, trip her up." I found not being able to read the words in the book or on the blackboard meant I had no idea what I was writing.

I kept it to myself. My parents did all they could to help me and would praise everything I did even if it was just learning a new word and spelling it or simply making it through another day without crying or wanting to give up. If only I had expressed my struggle and feelings they could have helped me conquer my fears and worries.

In middle school homework was introduced and at the end of the day you would need to fill in your homework diary. Just the thought of that blue book still gives me tiny butterflies. To start with, I copied words but when Dad read it he'd say, "What's this, my sweet?" I'd say I didn't know. I was then sat next to a boy who would help me by writing my homework down, but the kid was in such a rush every time that I could hardly read it and neither could Dad.   We came to the agreement that the teacher would write it down on paper for me to copy but I just took her writing back home.

So middle school was tough. It made me realise I was in real trouble. I had no way of asking for help because of peer pressure and older, different kids. I found that sometimes the words I wanted to use weren't always appropriate and the children around would look at me as if to say, "What's she talking about? She's obviously very special." I knew 'special' was an insult, not a compliment and it was heart breaking for me.

Chapter 3

Streams to cross

Although I learnt at middle school that my weaknesses were inside I discovered strength outside. This was PE. I found a joy in something I could do that didn't involve me having to write or read anything. I could just listen to the instructions and do it.

Another positive aspect was meeting a teacher called Mr Thompson.

When I started at middle school Mr Thompson called my parents in to talk to them about my progress and how I needed serious help. He suggested forgetting doing GCSE's and to just concentrate on here and now as I was so far behind. My parents were upset but glad he was willing to help me.

He was an amazing man who did everything he could to encourage me by letting me learn in a small class with lots of support. I remember the colourful posters explaining sums and shapes in maths and difficult words in English with times tables playing in the background. I think there must have been up to five or six of us in that classroom just sitting there absorbing everything that he was teaching us and the little tricks you can use to get over the problems. It was absolutely fantastic.
There was always an occasion where I would achieve something and Mr Thompson would say, "That's amazing!" and I would get a certificate or he would encourage me to tell one of the deputy heads. My parents were so proud of me, even with the tiniest thing and I would get first choice of our Friday night doughnut treat!

It was at this point the word dyslexia was used in front of me for the first time and explained. I was very upset one day in class because I didn't understand why I couldn't make sense where everyone else seemed to have no difficulty. Mr Thompson asked what the problem was. I explained through tears and that was when he slowly described what dyslexia was in a very simple way:

'When you look at a page do you see a lot of letters that make no sense or do you see words and meaning?'

"I just panic and see letters all over the page,'" I sobbed.

"That's dyslexia and that's why I'm here to help you."

He made it seem so simple. Now I had a label for what was going on but this just upset me and made me feel marked for life.

However, with Mr Thompson's help, I achieved more and, little by little, I moved back into mainstream and, with the support of lots of helpful teaching assistants, made my way through middle school.

Finally, there were the dreaded SATS where I was literally sick but I managed to scrape through on the second time round so I was on my way to upper school.

Chapter 4

My compass has gone missing

Upper school was a whole new ball game. To start with it wasn't too bad. I had already been through that terrifying first day phase and had people I could go to school with so I actually enjoyed my first day. I wasn't bothered I didn't look as cool as the other kids. I also discovered there was a safe place to go, a classroom with a lovely lady called Mrs Burns and teaching assistants who were really encouraging. That was until that first Science lesson.

I can still smell the Science room now. We sat there round the table that had the sink in the middle and tubes where you put the Bunsen burner on. The support teacher was sitting next to me and we had a text book all about atoms and particles. We all had to read aloud a part of this book and I whispered to the TA that I didn't want to read. She reassured me that she would sort it out. When my turn arrived I shook my head to the teacher but he said, "No, you need to read this." I said very quietly, "I can't."

The other children were beginning to mutter and I was so embarrassed and felt completely worthless. I looked at the TA and she said, "Just try a little bit". Again I mumbled that I didn't want to. Then the teacher said, "You need to read the next bit or do I need to pass it on to someone else who can read?"

I just felt like I wanted the floor to swallow me up. At that moment it felt like the worst day of my life.

Unfortunately, there were more days like that to come but I learnt to have an attitude. The more terrible I felt, the ruder I became. I realise now how difficult it was for the teachers but all I wanted was help and no one seemed to understand or be interested.

Chapter 5

Where's the summit?

Coming up to the GCSE year was another crucial point for me. I'd made it right through school, got my own little group of friends, my own little crazy nickname and, with help from my parents who were often as bewildered as me, I'd survived this far.

I had to do lots of revision which I did mainly at school because when I got home I needed a safe school- free zone. The GCSE's were not as terrifying as I thought they would be as I was given extra help.

Sometimes I had to just guess and did 'ip dip sky blue' with my eyes closed to find an answer on the multiple choice – any would do. For most of the exams I was able to go into a side room instead of having to be in the hall which was fantastic for me because it gave me more time to concentrate and think about what I was doing.

With the lessons I did enjoy like RE I did quite well because I was brought up in a Christian background so I knew many of the answers. One of the questions was on baptism and I was actually going through the process at the time so I could write really confidently. I also knew quite a lot about other cultures because I listened in the lessons so I managed to get myself a good grade for that. The other lesson was drama. Everyone loved being a bit of a drama queen and I was no exception. Drama was my way of being able to bring out the inner emotional child in me that was being trapped by horrible words and horrible lessons. I could express myself and I could be this person who could succeed and I got a good grade.

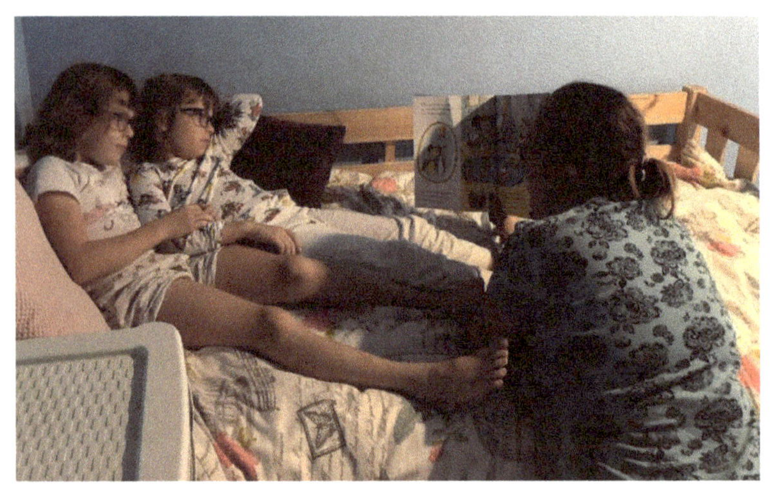

Chapter 6

The view's getting better

After I came out of the torture chamber called school I had the choice of staying on or going to college. Not surprisingly, I decided to go to college. I joined a group which was fantastic for people who were dyslexic and disabled.

The course was called Springboard. It seemed much easier for me: people were kinder and everyone was having difficulty. We were all in the same boat as we all struggled to read and we all struggled socially.

All the kids at college were great. I met some right characters there and I also learnt lots of different skills. I picked up some hospitality, a little bit of catering and I also learnt sign language. I had a great group of friends who I really could say were my friends, who I could actually call in the street and they would turn and say, "Look, there's Sarah." It was fantastic.

Chapter 7

More peaks ahead

Now the scary world of work called me to join it even if it was only part-time for now while I was at college. This was going to be a long and hard journey.

My first job was as a pharmacy assistant but it only lasted three months because, surprise, surprise, I struggled with the paperwork. I left there and joined Matalan but in these two processes I needed to fill in a paper application form. What I did was sit down with Dad and look at the questions. Then we wrote the answer out on a piece of paper; this was so frustrating but eventually two and a half hours later I had filled it in. It was easy at Matalan because it was just scanning items. If there were any issues I could just talk to management so that job lasted a year.

Tesco's was my next adventure and I lasted 18 months there. They were great at recognising and supporting my dyslexia. I worked in the café and they helped me with the recipe cards which had pictures and words so I could follow them in order to help the customers. I also met new friends who helped me survive by teaching me tricks of the trade like recognising pictures on the till. I think I only mischarged people a few times – every little helps!

Chapter 8

This isn't so bad!

Now my pockets were fuller I had some fun. I got myself a scooter! It was a Piaggio 125cc. It was royal blue and I loved it! I got through the practical test which was hard but educational so I had myself a set of wheels for my second year of college and I didn't need to rely on my parents any more. I had a new freedom, I could go anywhere. However, there was another hill to climb: THE HIGHWAY CODE. It was a huge struggle with lots of strange words and signs to work out but, with help from my family, and many arguments I managed to get through by the skin of my teeth.

Getting to places was another challenge. I couldn't read the place names so I always had to make sure I went with someone or remembered landmarks. Once, when I went to my sister's house, I ended up going the wrong way up a one way street and took two hours to complete a one hour journey. I arrived a blubbering mess. My Dad would make me map read in the car if we were going to London. He'd highlight the route because I couldn't read the place names. Salisbury and Durrington still crop up in my nightmares and it was the big M sign that helped me recognise Fleet.

Chapter 9

No ups without downs

Now in my twenties and with no wish to be with children but an even stronger wish to get away from Tesco's, I took a job in a nursery. Once there I started to enjoy the mess, the giggles and the wonderful uniqueness of each child. But there was one big thing that held me back: reading to the children was just too much of a struggle. I dreaded it although I really wanted to be able to do it.

The staff suggested I took books home to try but I was too embarrassed to do this. I wish I had now but it just didn't seem possible. As time went on we started to have to fill in forms to track children's development and this is where it all went terribly wrong for me. I would make spelling mistakes and couldn't make sense of what was written. They offered to help me but didn't actually do anything concrete. Hearing other staff say "don't give it to her, she won't be able to read it" or "that's definitely her, it's her spelling" are phrases I haven't forgotten. Then I was called into the office and reprimanded for my paperwork. Next was a verbal warning and it was downhill all the way from there until I left.

Chapter 10

Camping isn't fun

Now pregnant, paperwork continued to be my nightmare and lead to all sorts of problems. Reading about how to help my children grow inside me, what was the best pain relief and what were the best foods for pregnancy were all worries for me and would keep me up at night.

Maternity pay was not enough to survive with just my wage and my husband preferred spending to earning. Debt crept in and then there was all the paperwork that followed it which I couldn't keep on top of.

When we split up I had to climb Kilimanjaro all by myself – that's what it felt like. I had to set up my new flat and didn't have a clue how to change address, get all the appliances started, sort out the rent, pay the bills – I didn't know where to start. Dad would step in but it was often too late.

Chapter 11

There's never just one mountain

My reading got worse because I didn't use it; I could read a little bit but not enough. I was ashamed of myself because I didn't read and more embarrassed that I didn't understand. The girls were getting to an age where they wanted Mummy to read to them or take them to the library.

Oh, the library, that was like going back to school. Why would I want to go to a library? Books, words, argh! I didn't mind simple picture books with one word on each page but when it came to reading anything more, I wanted to throw the book away. The worst were names and surnames that writers thought would be fun for children but were a nightmare for me like Mrs Floppywoppybottom or even Cinderella. I would ask them to go to Nanny and Grandad. It was heart breaking not being able to read to your own children. I so wanted to sit and snuggle and have that motherly bond with them.

One of my main frustrations was not being able to teach the girls about everything around us from books. I thought I would love the worlds that encyclopaedias opened up but I didn't have a clue what the text said.

Also I wanted to be able to read them funny stories and do voices but that was impossible for me. The only stories I could feel safe with they were bored of. There are only so many hundred times you can read The Gruffalo or Each Peach Pear Plum. Books I knew were alright b u t new books were a whole different ball game. I would get all flustered and frustrated and end up turning the Disney Junior channel all the time because it was the only way of stopping them from asking me to read.

Sometimes when they asked me something, I would say I didn't know and I would change the subject.

Chapter 12

New equipment awaits

The government said that as a single parent you needed to attend a work force interview to access training and choices of career.

I thought this wouldn't lead to anything but in fact my coach was lovely. When I first met Carol she was so encouraging and made me feel wanted. She empowered me by using positive words and telling me, "You can do it." She asked me if there were any skills I'd like to pick up on and I mentioned cooking to start with. Then she offered me social groups I could go to and then suddenly I couldn't hold myself back. I could feel myself swallow the lump in my throat and blurted out: "I would desperately like to be able to read to my children."

I felt quite heartbroken having to admit the terrible word dyslexia to this woman who I feared was looking down her nose at me. But as I looked up she had a glisten in her eyes as if to say 'you poor love' and she gave me this sheet that said Read Easy on it. I just thought oh, another piece of useless paper to pile up on my kitchen table.

All I had to do was ring this woman up. It sounded so simple but it was such a big task. At the job centre if I had been given the option there and then I would have done it more quickly. Instead, I left it to be lost or drawn on as scrap on my kitchen table. Dad came to visit and found the leaflet. When he asked what it was I had no excuse left. I looked at it for a good solid hour and thought what am I doing? I said to myself if I don't do this now I never will. I picked up the telephone and I dialled the number. Then I cancelled it, redialled it, cancelled it, redialled it and cancelled it again. "Just do it, Sarah!" instructed Dad, sternly. I dialled the number and I got through to this lovely lady called Jenny.

Chapter 13

New boots, warm red scarf

"Um….er…I was given a sheet a paper," I stammered, not knowing what to say next. A very calm voice said, "It's Jenny from Read Easy." I felt myself blushing, not knowing what to say. "How did you hear about us?" she said in a kind, gentle voice. I told her about the job centre and then got a bit tearful – should I be admitting to someone else I couldn't read?

"You've called the right number; this is just what we're here for – to help people struggling with reading."

She went on to say, "Shall we meet up? Then we could do an assessment to see how you're getting on and what we can do to help you." My stomach tightened and I thought, that's it, I'm done for. Jenny arranged a time and a date. She said, "When you first meet me I will be wearing my red scarf. That's how you will know who I am." That wonderful red scarf!

As soon as I put the phone down negative thoughts got hold of me. What had I done, what mess was I in now? I had nightmares about turning up and finding a glamorous model in a red scarf pointing and laughing at me.

Somehow I got to where we were going to meet. I always get to places early because I like to make sure I have time to think about what's happening. As it got to just near the time I began to think she's not coming, this is all a joke, it's one big scam. Then I saw something red out of the corner of my eye and I realised this lady was coming towards me with a big smile on her face. She was wearing a red scarf!

"Hello, I'm Jenny, you must be Sarah."   I felt a strange combination of huge anxiety and huge relief. Then I started to feel trapped even though I stood outside in the street and at any point I could have run if I'd wanted to and not gone through with this. Instead I followed Jenny through some doors. As I stepped up the stairs my hands began to shake and get sweaty slipping off the bannisters. Jenny told the ladies at the top where we were going to before we went into a small room and sat down.

We had a little chat and she told me all about Read Easy. I wasn't really listening because I was so nervous and so uptight.

All I could think was how am I going to do this? How do I escape? I kept looking out of the window and checking the time. Then she brought out this piece of paper. I thought, that's it, I'm signing my life away and never going to be able to do anything again. It was a sheet which had lots of words on.

"I need you to have a look at these words," she said. "No pressure but can you go past these words one by one and tell me what they say and when you get to a word which you can't read, just skip over it and go to where you can." I went through the first side and then turned it over. Then I started to get nervous and wanted to cry. Jenny said, "That's it, that's enough, that's all I needed. You are fantastic. Well done, you have made the right choice, the first step. I am really proud of you."

To hear a stranger say they were proud of me made me think, hang on a minute, she might not be taking the mick, she might actually be able to help me.

Chapter 14

Warm cabin with my own St Bernard's

When I started with Read Easy they were very caring and wanted to find just the right reading partner for me. I had a couple of coaches who boosted my confidence and said, "You can do it, you are who you are."

One of my first coaches was called Phoebe and was such an inspiration. She was always enthusiastic, great fun and made me want to come back for more. We played lots of games like Bananagrams and Word Snap.

We read special books from the library too. I always remember The Frog in the Blender – yes, it was as disgusting as it sounds! Seeing my progress through the books and feeling someone believed in me made it worthwhile. We had lots of laughs and I felt comfy for the first time breaking down words and understanding how they worked. Using the little whiteboard Phoebe brought with her helped me expand my knowledge of all sorts of words. She knew my strengths and weaknesses and my concentration levels so she never pushed me further than I could go.

Little by little I became more confident. I found getting to grips with phonics began to open my eyes to what I had been missing. I felt bolder and braver. Who was going to stop me from picking up a book now and reading aloud? Yes, I made mistakes but who doesn't?

My parents backed me up all the way, encouraging me and telling me how proud they were of me.

Chapter 15

Telling my tale

Just as I was getting to the end of 18 months with Yes, We Can Read I was offered the opportunity to be filmed for Project Literacy to promote International Literacy Day.

This was going to involve a profile of me on a website and a video interview. I was filled with a mixture of pride and dread. I couldn't believe this was happening to me. I got miked up, had my hair and make- up done and sat with Phoebe to answer lots of questions. We were in the Grosvenor Hotel in Shaftesbury who had kindly lent us different rooms to read and film in. The director kept shouting at the kitchen staff to keep quiet!

I thought I'd feel petrified but in fact I found it so natural it was almost like I was just having a casual chat. I didn't want it to stop. When I look back at the footage each time I feel so proud of myself . What a change from all the self-criticism.

When I got my certificate 21 months after I started I felt over the moon, especially at the presentation with the cake! I got to meet the Chair of Read Easy too which was a privilege and an honour. I was making a step into the future; I was helping myself, not fighting any longer. I was also helping other people who struggle and I didn't want it to stop!

Chapter 16

Reflecting on the landscape

So now it was 2017 – what had changed for me in the last 2 years with Read Easy?

In 2015 I wouldn't dare pick up a book or attempt to read an email. I was way below where you should be when you leave school. I was miserable and felt like I was trapped in a mind prison because I didn't know how to express or explain myself. Wherever I could I stuck with easy things. My coach remembers me creeping into sessions like a little mouse and now says my head is held high.

In 2017 I felt confident in myself, not a failure and happy to ask for help. I wasn't ashamed if there were words that were still difficult to read to the girls. I could even ask them for help. Stop, think, take a deep breath – thanks, girls!

Chapter 17

New horizons ahead of me

But what now? When I finished I was a bit lost – where should I go from here? Then Jenny came to the rescue again. She suggested Moving Ahead, the next stage after Yes, We Can Read. I was bit wary of starting this because new experiences usually make me want to run away but then I realised I wanted not only to read but to write.

Jenny set up a meeting with Read Easy's literacy coordinator and we worked on a plan of what I wanted to learn. The thought of meeting a new coach terrified me. How was she (I'd already said I didn't want a male coach) going to judge me? That was always my fear when I met someone new.

Then I met Julia for the first time. I liked the fact that she was calm and quiet and listened. This helped me settle in quickly and take things at my own pace. The first time we had a lesson she gave me time to voice my concerns and worries.

And so the journey began again but from a new start. We started with punctuation and poems! There were lots of word puzzles and I even managed some crosswords which had always terrified me before. It felt like I could do lots and it brought back lots of things I realised I did know but I had forgotten.

After a couple of months of going over the basics I decided I'd like to write a book for children to help families who were going through the same problems I had struggled with. This led to a few false starts with trying to adapt fairy tale formats before I started writing about my own journey with dyslexia because, after all, that's what I knew best.

My wonderful coach, Julia, has listened and made it easy for me to understand literacy and helped me write this book. I couldn't believe I would be able to do it but it has chased those ghosts of the past far far away. The process has even helped with other personal issues, not directly but by giving me more headspace and confidence each time I write. And all the way through my ability to read and write has developed and been on show.

Chapter 18

Kind questions instead of harsh words

However, I'm charging ahead because just before Moving Ahead started something unexpected happened. International Literacy Day 2017 had gone so well I was offered the chance to go onto the Victoria Derbyshire Show. I was booked to talk to her co-host about my journey and struggles, how they have affected me as a person and a parent and how I'd come out the other side with the help of Read Easy.

I had never been on TV before. It was the chance of a lifetime. I was offered the opportunity to talk about me and all the things I'd experienced, most of which I've described here already. I felt like a voice for the dyslexic nation who normally had no voice. It was a huge honour to be picked because as a child I was never picked for anything.

Coming up to International Literacy Day 2018 the following year, the opportunity was offered to me again, but this time on Sky News! I couldn't believe the phone call inviting me, it was so awesome. This time I had to go to London the day before on my own as no one was available to come with me. I had to sort out the right train, walk to the hotel from the station (which included getting lost and unlost), book in (plenty of forms) and then decipher the menu in the hotel restaurant in dim lighting. Then I had to prepare to get myself up for 4.45 am!

I got to the Sky studio without problems and then had to book in again – more paperwork. I had layers of make-up plastered on and my trademark blue bow attached. As I got nearer to the studio

I had no idea what I was going to say and my stomach was churning but as soon as I sat down and they started talking to me all my fears disappeared. I felt completely at ease and the words flowed. I was able to express myself in a whole new manner; I felt like an adult for once. I was able to describe how Read Easy had transformed me from a grumpy caterpillar to a beautiful butterfly.

Chapter 19

A partner in climb

Jon has been such a positive part of my recent journey, encouraging me and praising me which fills me with a pride and passion to keep going forward. I need to include Jon in my story because he is very important. Before I didn't have the encouragement and help that he gives me. Previous partners have insulted me or knocked me down and treated me like a child with words like "really you're an adult, just pull yourself together" or nicknaming me nasty names.

This has all changed with Jon and his family who completely accept me for who I am and not my labels.

Chapter 20

Let's raise a glass

Now I can help others to read. I can encourage my children to never give up. I can stand proud of my achievements and say, yes, I am dyslexic but there will be no going back to a time when I found reading difficult.

Every time Read Easy mentions me as a success story I feel uplifted and always grateful to them.

Recently I moved house. As I was clearing the wardrobe I found dusty children's books that I had hidden down the back so I wouldn't have to read them. Now they are snuggle story time books, especially Mrs Vicar's Knickers!

I hope you enjoy reading this book as much as I have enjoyed writing it. I would like to give a special thanks to all the team at Read Easy, my parents and partner Jon and, of course, my children, Izzy and Betty who have inspired me to make this journey.

About Read Easy

Read Easy is a not-for-profit organisation that recruits, trains and supports volunteers to give one-to-one coaching to adults who struggle with reading. Working through community-based volunteer groups, Read Easy offers a free, friendly, flexible approach to learning to read for any adult who can't read at all, or who lacks confidence with reading.

Its success is founded on a one-to-one approach, using a highly effective, phonics-based reading scheme, supported by other learning activities. It gives people the opportunity to work in private and at their own pace and builds reading skills, confidence and self-esteem.

Most of us take our ability to read for granted and are unaware that there are around 2.4 million adults around us in the UK who either can't read at all or struggle with this most basic requirement for everyday life.

For more information go to: readeasy.org.uk.

To hear Sarah talking about her experiences just go to
https://readeasy.org.uk/testimonial/sarahs-story